yogawisdom

daily
inspiration
from
yoga
masters

yogawisdom

edited by
CASSANDRA POWERS

THE LYONS PRESS
GUILFORD, CONNECTICUT

An imprint of The Globe Pequot Press

The Lyons Press is an imprint of The Globe Pequot Press.

DESIGN BY CLAIRE ZOGHB

ISBN 1-58574-709-2

Printed in the United States of America

10 9 8 7 6 5 4 3 2 1

Library of Congress Cataloging-in-Publication data is available
on file.

for my aunt susie

acknowledgments

No creative endeavor, great or small, is a solitary one. I would like to thank the following people for their help: my editors, Ann Treistman and Holly Rubino, for their trust and enthusiasm; John M. Lundquist and Gamil Youssef of the Asian and Middle Eastern Division at the New York Public Library for their interest and patience; and the rest of the staff who helped me so much: Professor Gary A. Tubb of Columbia University for his expertise; all the good people at Center for Yoga in Los Angeles; and, from the bottom of my heart, my parents, whose blind faith in me is the greatest gift I know.

contents

introduction

THE ANCIENT PHYSICAL AND SPIRITUAL DISCIPLINE of yoga offers a way to open the closed places within ourselves, from a stiff hip making a hike uncomfortable to an ingrained mind-set that binds us to bad habits. Like so many Americans, I am fascinated by the concept of reinvention. This potential within yoga to initiate change, I believe, is the reason we are drawn to it. Change is as close as we can get to drinking from the Holy Grail, and in this spirit, we ask yoga to help us uncover a new self, a new life.

When I began yoga, my motive was far shallower! All the people I knew who did yoga looked young for their age. I still believe this to be true, even after plenty of time to contemplate yoga's more sublime offerings. The key is flexibility of both mind and body. Think of someone old, and what do you see? Restricted movement, weak muscles, perhaps a stubborn attitude. Yoga stretches and strengthens all aspects of the human body and soul. Our minds can go beyond our opinions, our bodies become confident with new-found agility.

Yoga is hot almost everywhere now, but it is especially sizzling in Los Angeles. This city invents a new style of yoga with almost the same rapidity as it discovers a new star. Because of this, LA is a fun place to experiment. I had practiced yoga before I moved to LA, but I had never been immersed. Fresh off the freeway from Vermont, I decided to apply for a job in a yoga studio. Immersion I got. What an introduction to Hollywood, for yoga studio culture and Hollywood life are close to synonymous these days. Maybe it's the unpredictable lifestyle of trying to make it in Tinseltown that has created a rush on yoga. While I encountered plenty of ironies and hypocrisies—Angelenos vie for mat space the same way they compete for parking on Sunset—I was surrounded by people with a genuine interest in and knowledge of yoga, which piqued my curiosity. My interest grew in direct proportion to how good yoga made me feel. While it may sound hokey, completing a yoga class consistently left me feeling relaxed, refreshed, and more tolerant of everyday annoyances. Yes, I'm a mat snob and tote my own rather than use communal ones, but I'm better able to take a deep breath if someone cuts me off on the freeway. My increased flexibility, in my attitude as much as my hamstrings, is far more rewarding than my fastest mile ever was.

While yoga has evolved, incredibly, certain themes still resonate. The eight limbs of yoga, as set forth by Patanjali, link the many offshoots and schools of thought that exist. The eight limbs are:

- *Yama* (Discipline), which involves being good to others
- *Niyama* (Personal Purity), being good to oneself
- *Asana* (Posture), practicing different poses for the purpose of detoxing and preparing the body for deep meditation
- *Pranayama* (Breath), breathing with awareness for cleansing
- *Pratyahara* (Withdrawal of the Senses), letting go of attachment to the material world

- *Dharana* (Concentration), focusing,
  perhaps on a mantra
- *Dhyana* (Meditation), releasing
  stray thoughts
- *Samadhi* (Divine Union), superconsciousness of and union with Brahman, the
  divine essence of all that we know and
  do not know

These concepts form the core of yogic teachings, and instructors still learn about them during
their training. I have edited this book so that the
entries follow the arc of the eight limbs. One important note: while the eight limbs are always listed
in particular order, they are not levels or steps in the
sense that one moves from one level to the next, like
a beginner moves on to intermediate. All the limbs
are equal, and do not fall away as you progress.

As I learned to navigate LA's freeways, I also struggled to unravel the many strands of yoga. Culling quotes on yoga helped to sort out the maze of thoughts, impressions, and beliefs that insulate the core truths. The purpose of a collection of quotes is twofold. The first is to gather nuggets of truth that can help us understand what yoga is, and the second is to give a sense of the range of thinking on yoga—you'll find overlaps as well as contradictions among sources. Collected here are the words of ancient masters like Patanjali as well as the modern interpretations of scholars and instructors like Georg Feuerstein and Donna Farhi. My hope is that these quotes may help to inform and inspire your practice. Sometimes, when we do things repeatedly, we forget why we do them. Whether you do asanas each day, or evening meditation, or whether you focus on taking deeper breaths when you can, I hope

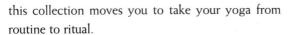
this collection moves you to take your yoga from routine to ritual.

As we explore the eight limbs through the written word and then practice, yoga becomes more than a promise of a youthful body. Yoga is the quest for meaning. It is an ancient response to the human need to answer questions about our place and purpose in the universe. Staying lean and flexible may be the goals that bring us to yoga, but the possibility of unlocking our innermost mysteries brings our whole self to the endeavor, our bodies serving as gateways to enlightenment.

Whether or not you ever reach superconsciousness isn't the point; neither is it forcing your body into alarming postures. When we let go of our notions of result, that is yoga. When we free ourselves of the need to excel, that also is yoga. When we genuinely wish to unite our scattered thoughts and passions with a power beyond ourselves, that, in-deed, is yoga.

Namaste.

NOTE: Many of the sources for the following quotes are old. Their emphasis on the male point of view is a function of their eras, and are quoted here because of their intrinsic thoughtfulness.

yogawisdom

LIMBS 1 AND 2

embracing the discipline of kindness to others and to ourselves

YAMAS | NIYAMAS

YAMAS: *nonviolence, nonstealing, chastity, absence of greed, truthfulness*

NIYAMAS: *purity, contentment, austerity, study of sacred texts, awareness of divine*

Committing to these principles is not so much about rigidity and rules as it is about leading a life free from negative energy. The way to divine consciousness begins with purity in body, mind, and deed.

∞

"We are responsible for what we are; and whatever we wish ourselves to be, we have the power to make ourselves."

—SWAMI VIVEKANANDA

"Life is not inherently meaningful. We *make* meaning happen through the attention and care we express through our actions."

—DONNA FARHI

"The aim of yoga is to eliminate the control that material nature exerts over the human spirit, to rediscover through introspective practice what the poet T. S. Eliot called 'the still point of the turning world.'"

—BARBARA STOLER MILLER

"When people have desires, it is like trees having insects; consumed within unknown, before long they collapse."

—THOMAS CLEARY

"We must remember that nothing in this world really belongs to us. At best, we are merely borrowers."

—CHRISTOPHER ISHERWOOD

"Perfect happiness is attained through contentment."

—PATANJALI, 42, PART 2

∞

"My friend, if you study human nature carefully, you will find that nobody is low and nobody is high. It is true that there is a realm of darkness and above it, a realm of light, but the dwellers in this region of light are neither high nor low—they are transcendent."

—SHRI DADA SANGHITA

"A yogi must avoid the two extremes of luxury and austerity."

—SWAMI VIVEKANANDA

"Today, we tend to live mainly on the surface of our existence. We are busy with changing objects and events. We identify with these changes. . . . We are slaves to those changes."

—SWAMI CHINMAYANANDA

"Few of us can reach profound and perfect enlightenment in profound and perfect isolation."

—KATE WHEELER

"But such a tiny and trivial thing as an umbrella can deprive you of the sight of such a stupendous fact as the sun."

—MEHER BABA

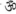
"Yoga is not about self-improvement, it's about self-acceptance."

—GURMUKH

"You may fancy you are in a free state but no transformation is real which is not reflected in your conduct."

—VIMALA THAKAR

"The practice of Yoga brings us face to face with
the extraordinary complexity of our own being."
—SRI AUROBINDO

"As a fire is obscured by smoke,
as a mirror is covered by dust,
as a fetus is wrapped in its membrane,
so wisdom is obscured by desire."
—*BHAGAVAD GITA*, 3.38

"Wealth and happiness do not dwell together."
—Swami Venkatesananda

"The Yogi knows that the paths of ruin or of salvation lie within himself."
—B. K. S. Iyengar

"The ego is like a rock projecting out of a river. It creates resistance and causes the otherwise peaceful flow of the water to form eddies and cross currents."

—GEORG FEUERSTEIN

"We each need to make peace with our own memories. We have all done things that make us flinch."

—LAMA SURYA DAS

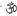
"I find that so many people are doing this in their yoga practice and probably in every aspect of their lives—they're always trying to do their life right."

—RODNEY YEE

"Verbal knowledge is not adequate to destroy the delusions of the worldly rounds. By mere talk of the lamp the darkness does not recede."

—KULARNAVA, 1.97

"You might say that we use ourselves to discover ourselves."

—JUDITH LASATER

∞

"Two distinct paths are open to us, the path of the good and the path of the pleasant."

—SWAMI CHINMAYANANDA

"When you dwell on yourself, preoccupied with private profit and personal pleasure, you lose your resilience. A little knock at the door explodes like a pistol shot."

—EKNATH EASWARAN (1992)

∞

"To experience true creativity, we must always be willing to let go of the results, whether it's a novel or our children."

—GURMUKH

"For those with preferences,
suffering is inevitable."
—THAI MONK

"Where there is the 'I' there is bondage,
where there is no 'I' there is release."
—*ASHTAVAKRA GITA*, 8.4 (STEPHEN CROSS)

"The most positive action we can perform to contribute to the momentous task of bringing our planet back into balance is to start changing ourselves."

—SWAMI VISHNU-DEVANANDA

"Looking outside ourselves for wholeness brings disappointment and pain. . . . As long as our male and female energies remain unbalanced, we remain desperate for the company of others to cease this indeterminate ache."

—LIZ LARK

"No matter how hard you pursue pleasure and success, there are times when you fail. No matter how fast you flee, there are times when pain catches up with you."

—BHANTE HENEPOLA GUNARATANA

"Everything comes to pass, nothing comes to stay."

—MATTHEW FLICKSTEIN

"Freedom is not worth having if it does not connote freedom to err."

—GANDHI

"You have the privilege and choice to make your own heaven right here; you have all the means to do so."

—PARAMAHANSA YOGANANDA (1999)

"We should know who we are and how we relate to other people. That is not easy, for we do not have such a clear mirror for our minds as we do for our bodies."

—T. K. V. DESIKACHAR

∞

"For spiritual practice to develop, it is absolutely essential that we establish a basis of moral conduct in our lives."

—JOSEPH GOLDSTEIN AND
JACK KORNFIELD

"There is nothing wrong with having relationships and possessions. The problem is that we see them as having some inherent ability to satisfy us."
—KATHLEEN MCDONALD

"The price of peace includes the sacrifice of personal gains and ego pursuits for the greater good of spiritual unfoldment and natural evolution which will bring about Universal Peace."
—SWAMI GITANANDA

"The infinite has never abandoned its infinity."
—SWAMI VENKATESANANDA

"The real beginning of spiritual practice is evident when we accept responsibility for ourselves, that is, when we acknowledge that ultimately there are no answers outside of ourselves, and no gurus, no teachers, and no philosophies that can solve the problems of our lives."
—JUDITH LASATER

"This humanity is the honey of all beings, and all beings are the honey of this humanity."

—*Brhadaranyaka Upanishad*, 2.5.14

"Body consciousness is a snake and physical comforts are its coils."

—Shri Dada Sanghita

"The tantric path is not without pitfalls, because passion becomes an obstacle for one who does not have purity of heart and mind."

—MIRANDA SHAW

"Whether we realize it or not, our minds are hypnotized by the outer world, captured by these exterior needs and desires."

—GURUDEV SHREE CHITRABHANU

"In this century we have made remarkable material progress, but basically we are the same as we were thousands of years ago. Our spiritual needs are still very great."

—HIS HOLINESS THE DALAI LAMA
(MARGARET GEE)

∞

"The basic issue of human suffering including moral, religious and psychological problems has been traced to one ultimate cause, to wit, self-estrangement, alienation from existence, loss of contact with Being."

—HARIDAS CHAUDHURI

"Most people brood on the past and do not know how to live here and now. That is the cause of their suffering."

—SWAMI RAMA

∞

"In this secular age great numbers of men and women make sex a substitute for religion and find in it a way of catching momentarily something of the non-duality, timelessness, and ego-oblitera- tion experienced by the mystics. . . . If men and women were granted the experience of orgasm only once or twice in their lives, one could well envisage a world religion being based on it."

—JAMES HEWITT

"Yoga is not a matter of suppressing the ego, or anything else for that matter, but of *transcending* it."
—GEORG FEUERSTEIN

∞

"As between individuals, so between cultures: real knowledge of the other, and thereby of oneself, arises and flourishes largely in a state of love."
—RAVI RAVINDRA

"Therefore superior people study the Way: they look upon merit and fame, wealth and status, as floating clouds, letting them go and come without being moved by them while in their very midst."

—THOMAS CLEARY

"It is valuable to go to the source, the master, but . . . if we are open, everyone we meet can be a guru. . . . Ultimately, we must inquire within."

—LIZ LARK

"If your words are not harnessed to purity of mind, they wander from door to door, and you never know what will become of them."

—SWAMI CHIDVILASANANDA

"Do not confuse relaxation with laziness or inertia."

—RICHARD HITTLEMAN

"Our lives are patterns of accumulation in which we are never still or at rest."
—DAVID FRAWLEY

∞

"Good and evil are like living organisms dwelling in the field of our mind and we nourish or starve them according to the value of our thoughts, words, and deeds."
—SHRI DADA SANGHITA

"The sound OM . . . is a giving and taking at the same time; a taking that is free from greediness and a giving that does not try to force gifts upon others."

— ANAGARIKA BRAHMACARI GOVINDA

"Thus, the Law of Karma, when properly understood, is a great vital force. It makes us the architects of our own future."

—SWAMI CHINMAYANANDA

"Dealing in words is more dangerous than playing with fire. Words have their own ways of intoxicating you."

—VIMALA THAKAR

"The silkworm makes its own cocoon, but does not know how to get out and consequently dies in it."

—RAMAKRISHNA

"Believing fundamentally that this life is the only one, modern people have developed no long term vision. So there is nothing to restrain them from plundering the planet for their own immediate ends and from living in a selfish way that could prove fatal for the future."

—SOGYAL RINPOCHE

"Repression forces your mind to be more deeply entrenched in those things from which you are trying to escape."

—VIMALA MCCLURE

"In your very imperfections you will find the basis for your firm way-seeking mind."

—SHUNRYO SUZUKI

"I sit at my window gazing
The world passes by, nods to me
And is gone."

—TAGORE

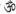
"The Yamas and Niyamas are there to help us work out how we live our yoga while we live with others."

—VALERIE JEREMIJENKO

∞

"You seek too much information and not enough transformation."

—SAI BABA

"Is there no art which could enable us to pass through the sense and object relationships without parting with the tenderness and elasticity of childhood?"

—VIMALA THAKAR

"The whole search for enlightenment is to seek within, to become aware that you are complete in yourself."

—SWAMI RAMA

"An enlightened . . . person *has* an emotion, but does not *become* the emotion."

—SWAMI CHINMAYANANDA

"Dispassion is the sign of mastery over the craving for sensuous objects."

—PATANJALI, 15, PART 1

(BARBARA STOLER MILLER)

"We feed on the world in increasingly desperate attempts to compensate for feelings of incompleteness, separation, and alienation."
—KEN MCLEOD

"Desire is endless."
—DAININ KATAGIRI

"The western mind is linear, the eastern mind is circular. So in the east a lover can wait."

—BHAGWAN SHREE RAJNEESH

"I adore myself.
How wonderful I am!"

—*ASHTAVAKRA GITA*

"Tantra represents the endeavor to penetrate the
mystic link between the finite and the infinite,
the individual and the cosmos. Whilst to some,
whatever is spiritual may seem to exclude that
which is earthly, both are harmoniously recon-
ciled in Tantra."

—SWAMI PARITOSANANDA AND
VISHWARUPANANDA

∞

"Death does not wait to see if things are done or
not done."

—*KULARNAVA*, 1.42

"Experiences are temporary; the goal of *kaivalya* (liberation) is permanent."

—SARASVATI BUHRMAN

"It's not the actual enlightenment experience alone that counts, but the living of it, embodying it . . . working out its implications in everyday life. . . . True spiritual realization manifests as enlightened activity . . . Not just epiphanies. In the meantime, stay awake to what you are experiencing right now. It's the best show in town."

—LAMA SURYA DAS

"You can't change someone else, and even if you
. . . could, you would still be the main challenge
in your own life."

—GURMUKH

"To end this pervasive sorrow, as we all desire in
our heart of hearts, we have to disengage our
identity from nature and shift it to where it belongs, on the person. It's easier said than done."

—RICHARD ROSEN

"Spiritual progress is therefore not separated off from the body nor from desire, but these are gradually educated to renounce what harms them. To be sure, it is not a matter of renouncing for the sake of renouncing, but of renouncing what impedes . . . bliss in this life."

—LUCE IRIGARAY

"Do not cut off even a blade of grass uselessly."

—*KULARNAVA*, 5.46

"Yoga's metaphysics diagnoses the human condition as a state of suffering due to ignorance whose specific form is misidentification of the Self with materiality."

—GREGORY P. FIELDS

∞

"What else is left of a greedy man except a handful of ashes."

—SWAMI VENKATESANANDA

"All the problems that appear so immediate and important—like whether we will be loved or if our friends and family can be happy—are not the real issue and cannot be solved directly. The real issue is how to use the most important and central instrument in our lives—the mind itself."

—DAVID FRAWLEY

"This prison of mundane life rests on the central pillar of egoism."

—SWAMI BRAHMANANDA

"If man wants the happiness he is striving for, let him be more aggressive towards himself and more tolerant towards others."

—MEHER BABA

"I have a very simple philosophy about life. . . . Teach, preach and advocate Yoga which is Oneness. . . . Do not teach, preach or advocate Twoness. Therefore, friction, quarrels, the use of force, taking of drugs or the use of tobacco and alcohol are not allowed, for they all create a schism of one type or another. Those who still want these habits are welcome to them and should go back into the world for a few more Karmic lessons. . . . That's what the outer world is for."

—SWAMI GITANANDA

"We must remember that insecurity is not our in-born nature. It is a mental creation and an addiction born of our cultural programming."

—GURUDEV SHREE CHITRABHANU

"Life . . . is a reward, and it is given only to those . . . who deserve it. Now it is your right to enjoy; it will be a sin if you don't enjoy. . . . No, leave it a little happier, a little more beautiful, a little more fragrant."

—OSHO (1999)

"The mystics will tell us that when we have a desire for a certain . . . experience, and we fulfill that desire, the happiness we feel is not something given by that thing or that experience; it is due to having no craving for a little while."

—EKNATH EASWARAN (1993)

"All our lives we are engaged in preserving our experiences and keeping them fresh by artificially sprinkling the water of memory over them. They have ceased to retain their original smell and fragrance. Do you call it life—this effort at the preservation of a phantom freshness in something that is withered and gone?"

—VIMALA THAKAR

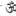
"Your loss is your gain."

—Nisargadatta Maharaj

"Tantra recognizes that we yearn to be happy and this desire drives all our actions. However, this grasping for pleasure keeps us swimming in an ocean of "samsara" (to circle) where we suffer a perpetual cycle of frustrations."

—Liz Lark

"We can travel a long way and do many things, but our deepest happiness is not born from accumulating new experiences. It is born from letting go of what is unnecessary."

—SHARON SALZBERG

∞

"The world will try to find fault with you. Do not mind its criticism but note carefully what your introspection reveals to you."

—SHRI DADA SANGHITA

"It is in a thousand and one bonds of loving rela-
tionship with fellow beings that true freedom is
to be enjoyed."

—HARIDAS CHAUDHURI

LIMB 3

purifying the body

ASANA

W E MAY KNOW THE THIRD LIMB OF ASANA BEST.
Originally referring to the seated meditation posture,
asana now envelops the many poses we do in a hatha yoga
class. Here, the aim is to link movement with breath in an
effort to still the mind. In addition, asanas work to wring
out toxins and balance the body's many chemical functions.
Now cleansed, we are ready for further communion with
Brahman. The more our bodies learn to release, the more re-
ceptive we are to the present moment, where truth resides.

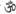
"The duality of sun and moon—or of bringing any opposites into balance—is at the root of Hatha Yoga."

—ILA AND DINABANDHU SARLEY

"All the eight limbs of yoga are in one pose."

—PATRICIA WALDEN

"Question: What does it mean to fail in yoga?
Maharaj: There can be no defeat in yoga. This
battle is always won, for it is a battle between the
true and the false. The false has no chance. . . . It
is like traveling a long and arduous road in an unknown country. Of all the innumerable steps
there is only the last which brings you to your
destination. Yet you will not consider all previous steps as failures."

—NISARGADATTA MAHARAJ

"Experience yourself in silence."

—ERICH SCHIFFMANN

"They are simply representatives of our own highest nature, that serve to evoke our own essential humanness."

—STEPHEN COPE, ON TEACHERS

∽

"When this body has been so magnificently and artistically created by God, it is only fitting that we should maintain it in good health and harmony by the most excellent and artistic science of Yoga."

—GEETA S. IYENGAR

"Asanas attune the body to meditation, just as a guitar is tuned."
—PARITOSANANDA AND
VISHWARUPANANDA

"We envy because we compare."
—JOHN MCAFEE

"The Surrender must be complete."
—SRI AUROBINDO

"Hatha Yoga helps us observe and learn about our bodies and minds as they are, without judgment."
—GRETCHEN ROSE NEWMARK

"What the mind has forgotten, the body remembers long after."
—LILIAS FOLAN

"In this world, there are two persons:
the transient and the eternal;
all beings are transient as bodies,
but eternal within the self."
—*Bhagavad Gita*, 15.16

∞

"Experience is the only teacher we have."
—Swami Vivekananda

"While performing asanas, the student's body assumes numerous forms of life found in creation . . . from the lowliest insect to the most perfect sage—and he learns that in all these breathes the same universal spirit."

—B. K. S. IYENGAR (1965)

∞

"The emphasis on *asana* practice is also specific to the age in which we live, for we live in a time of extreme dissociation from bodily experience."

—DONNA FARHI

"Yoga is essentially a practice for your soul, working through the medium of your body."
—TARA FRASER

∝

"While not wishing to under-value the importance of postural training and relaxation, it should be stressed that, in the opulent palace of hatha-yoga, these aspects constitute merely the gates at the entrance."
—MIKEL BURLEY

"My ashtanga practice has stagnated, backpedaled, inched forward, slid back, and blossomed so many times that I have jettisoned the notion of 'progress' so dear to my western conditioning."

—LOIS NESBITT

"So long as we are in conflict with our body, we cannot find peace of mind."

—GEORG FEUERSTEIN

"What we're trying to do in yoga is to create a union, and so to deepen a yoga pose is to actually increase the union of the pose, not necessarily put your leg around your head."
—RODNEY YEE

"A clean spirit must build a clean body."
—GANDHI

"I see exercise taking a perverted detour. . . . Now I see it as having nothing to do with health."

—BRYAN KEST

"What is the use of merely listening to lectures? The real thing is practice."

—RAMAKRISHNA

"Once you have begun to master the postures . . .
beware of excessive pride or ambition."
—TARA FRASER

∞

"The expression of the spirit increases in proportion to the development of the body and mind in which it is encased."
—SWAMI VISHNU-DEVANANDA

"Yoga's approach recognizes that the roots of mental problems are found on all levels of human existence: physical, mental, and spiritual, and only when all three levels are tended to can lasting mental health be attained."

—PARITOSANANDA AND
VISHWARUPANANDA

"Becoming obsessive about practicing is to be avoided because that can be another form of grasping or attachment."

—LIZ LARK

"The Body is the only means by which the soul manifests itself."

—GANDHI

∞

"Sthira is steadiness and alertness. Sukha refers to the ability to remain comfortable in a posture. Both qualities should be present to the same degree when practicing any posture."

—T. K. V. DESIKACHAR

"The places where you have the most resistance are actually . . . going to be the areas of greatest liberation."

—RODNEY YEE

"Every shape, every form, every hexagon and tri-angle, every object, everything that is experienced with the physical body, points to something finer within."

—PANDIT USHARBUDH ARYA

"The most tangible way that we can know what it means to be compassionate or not grasping is directly through the cellular experience of the body."
—DONNA FARHI

"Physical postures . . . are intended only for some bodily preparation entitling one to take up higher phases of yogic practice such as concentration, meditation, and the like."
—HARIDAS CHAUDHURI

"The yogi will tell you that you feel and look as young as your spine is elastic."
—RICHARD HITTLEMAN

"Ayurveda views the physical body as a crystallization of deep-seated mental tendencies carried over from previous lives."
—DAVID FRAWLEY

"The purpose and meaning of life can be found deep within the mystical meanings of the Hatha Yoga Asanas."

—SWAMI SIVANANDA RADHA

∞

"If there is any true temple . . . it is our own body."

—MAHARAJ CHARAN SINGH

"Your spiritual life does not depend on belief but on practice."

—VIMALA MCCLURE

"Having patience I should develop enthusiasm;
For awakening will dwell only in those who
    exert themselves.
Just as there is no movement without wind,
So merit does not occur without enthusiasm."

—ACHARYA SHANTIDEVA, 6.1,1

"The *asanas* are useful maps to explore yourself,
but they are not the territory."

—Donna Farhi

∞

"The Buddha . . . studied many religions, but he
was not satisfied with their practices. . . . He was
not interested in some metaphysical existence,
but in his own body and mind, here and now."

—Shunryo Suzuki

"If you are trying hard to relax, how can you be relaxed? You are too busy trying!"

—RICHARD HITTLEMAN

"Make it a way of life to observe yourself, for by being aware of your behavior you will be your own guru. "

—KEVIN AND VENIKA KINGSLAND

"I had always approached my body as if it were a problem needing to be solved. . . . But here I was, truly broken now, weak, emaciated, yet in front of me this teacher was saying that just by virtue of my being, I was complete. I always had been."
—SAMANTHA DUNN

"Any act, any movement of the body, is a dance. That becomes so not by attending a dance school, but by watching the mind watching the body."
—PANDIT USHARBUDH ARYA

"The physical practice of yoga is deeply anchored in me now that I know it more by its occasional absence."

—ALISON WEST

"Your burden is of false self-identifications— abandon them all."

—NISARGADATTA MAHARAJ

"In the Eastern tradition of teaching the aspirant is not 'spoon-fed' information, but rather is stimulated by the guru to be a discoverer, an adventurer, an investigator of his or her own body laboratory."

—SWAMI SIVANANDA RADHA

"Yoga is not a process of denial, but of revelation. . . . Our true spiritual nature exists. . . . All that we can do is clarify its existence, through the practice of yoga, and then honor it in the living of our lives."

—GODFREY DEVEREUX

"All Yoga is in its nature a new birth; it is a birth out of the ordinary."

—SRI AUROBINDO

"The greatest leverage for healing is found at the subtlest levels of function."

—RUDOLPH BALLENTINE

"Without discipline in spiritual pursuits, the central nervous system doesn't have a chance to adjust and grow with the increased demand. It would be like putting a high voltage into a small bulb—it is bound to explode."

—SWAMI SIVANANDA RADHA

"The body is no longer educated to develop its perceptions spiritually, but to detach itself from the sensible for a more abstract, more speculative, more sociological culture."

—LUCE IRIGARAY

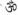
"Health . . . is not so much a *state*, but a *force*: the power to resist and overcome threats to one's well-being."

—GREGORY P. FIELDS

"When there is resistance in a yoga pose, it occurs because you have a mental concept of what you'd like the pose to be that is in conflict with what your body is capable of doing in that moment. But can you simply back up your expectations and be involved with what is happening right now? Isn't that enough?"

—RODNEY YEE

"Your positivity can become a castle around you which will protect you from the arrow of negativity."

—GURUDEV SHREE CHITRABHANU

"Enjoyment is just the sound of being centered."

—OSHO (1999)

"What kind of Yoga do you want to practice, the Yoga of getting or the Yoga of giving?"

—NISARGADATTA MAHARAJ

"Transformation can only take place immediately; the revolution is now, not tomorrow."

— J. KRISHNAMURTI

"Practicing yoga during the day is a matter of keeping your eyes on the road and one ear turned toward the infinite."

—ERICH SCHIFFMANN

∞

"We are aware of yoga only as a technique to gain . . . strength, flexibility, or increased health. And indeed these are potent side effects of the practice. But that is what they are: side effects. To focus on these largely insignificant manifestations is to miss the point entirely."

—JOHN MCAFEE

"I would like for people to realize that yoga is not about touching your toes."

—GARY KRAFSTOW

LIMB 4

breath control

PRANAYAMA

ORDINARILY, WE DON'T NOTICE OUR BREATH, AND yet it is our very essence. The secret of **Pranayama** is in its transformative powers. We neglect to tap into these powers because the breath silently takes care of itself. As the breath is a manifestation of prana, the life force in all, it provides the opportunity to unhinge our inherent capacity for calm enlightenment.

"We take over 24,000 breaths and exchange over 10,000 gallons of air in our lungs every day of our lives."

—RICHARD C. MILLER

"As a fire blazes brightly when the covering of ash over it is scattered by the wind, the divine fire within the body shines in all its majesty when the ashes of desire are scattered by the practice of pranayama."

—B. K. S. IYENGAR (1965)

"Breathing, according to me, corresponds to taking charge of one's own life."
—LUCE IRIGARAY

"Yogic breathing is not a competition to see how much air we can cram into our lungs."
— JAMES HEWITT

"Love more . . . that is breathing out . . . and your body will gather energy from the whole cosmos. You create the vacuum and the energy comes."
—BHAGWAN SHREE RAJNEESH

"In our uniquely human capacity to connect movement with breath and spiritual meaning, yoga is born."
—GURMUKH

"Grace is within you. If it were external,
it would be useless."

—SHRI RAMANA MAHARSI

"The harmonizing of opposing forces is a key
aspect of yoga—hot energy is united with cool
energy, strong with soft, and masculine with
feminine."

—TARA FRASER

"In all the yogas, we must be brave, because we are playing with fire—our energies, our potential, our shadows—channeling and sublimating them."

—LIZ LARK

"Breathing and speaking use breath in an almost inverse manner. . . . From this point of view it is interesting to note that people who do not breathe, or who breathe poorly, cannot stop speaking."

—LUCE IRIGARAY

"You can only have bliss if you don't chase it."
—BHANTE HENEPOLA GUNARATANA

∞

"Without proper breathing, the yoga postures are nothing more than calisthenics."
—RACHEL SCHAEFFER

∞

"We begin where we are and how we are, and whatever happens, happens."
—T. K. V. DESIKACHAR

"Everything is in the trying. It is no loss of merit when failure occurs . . . for by trying we learn."

—GAVIN AND YVONNE FROST

"They indeed are fools who are satisfied with the fruits of their past effort and do not engage themselves in self-effort now."

—SWAMI VENKATESANANDA

"As all the small rivulets flow into the sea, so should the attention point to the breath within."

—SWAMI NITYANANDA

"As all the spokes are fastened to the hub and the rim of a wheel, so to one's self (atman) are fastened all beings, all the gods, all the worlds, all the breaths."

—BRHADARANYAKA UPANISHAD, 2.5.15

"Prana is merely the life energy by which divinity brings into existence the organic kingdoms and acts on the organic structures, as it creates and acts on the universe by means of physical energy."

—GOPI KRISHNA

∞

"Yogic breathing is based on rhythm, and rhythm is life."

—JAMES HEWITT

"To live, work and suffer on this shore in faithfulness to the whispers from the other shore is spiritual life."

—Ravi Ravindra

"Human energy is always in communion with heaven and earth in the alternation of exhalation and inhalation."

—Thomas Cleary

"'If the breathing is at all unsettled, life is not your own.'"

—Qiu

∞

"Only when we are willing to give away every last particle of breath, which is our life force, can we truly receive."

—Gurmukh

"There is no fire without wind. . . . It is impossible to live even for five seconds without prana-vayu, the Breath of Life."

—SWAMI NITYANANDA

∞

"Breathing becomes a vehicle of spiritual experience, the mediator between body and mind."

—ANAGARIKA BRAHMACARI GOVINDA

"What we call 'I' is just a swinging door which moves when we inhale and when we exhale."
—SHUNRYO SUZUKI

"Pranayama . . . is a process of transforming our individual energy into cosmic energy."
—KEVIN AND VENIKA KINGSLAND

ॐ

"We come to this work because the alternative, being consumed by the effort to ignore the mystery of being, is no longer acceptable."
—KEN MCLEOD

∞

"If we want to know real spiritual life, we have to taste ourselves as we really are."
—DAININ KATAGIRI

"If it appears difficult, it is you who make it difficult. The great way is easy. . . . Even trees follow it, rivers follow it, rocks follow it. How can it be difficult? . . . and the trick to make any easy thing difficult is to choose, to make a distinction."

—BHAGWAN SHREE RAJNEESH

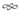

"Regular practice of pranayama is like putting money in the bank—it develops a reserve of health, energy, and vitality upon which we can draw long after we've finished our practice."

—RICHARD C. MILLER

"Sometimes there is a real pain in sitting, and sometimes the ego just tries to distract us by creating itches we will want to scratch."
—SARASVATI BUHRMAN

"The Yogi's life is not measured by the number of his days but by the number of his breaths."
—B. K. S. IYENGAR (1965)

"Life is happiness and unhappiness. Life is day and night, life is life and death. You have to be aware of both."

—OSHO (1999)

∞

"In real experiencing, real experimentation, there cannot be the search for the result."

—J. KRISHNAMURTI

"Through practicing breathing . . . I learned . . . the body is the site of the incarnation of the divine and I have to treat is as such."

—LUCE IRIGARAY

∞

"There is nothing we need to be whole that does not already exist within us."

—JUDITH LASATER

"There's so much to let go of isn't there? Your nostalgia and your regrets. Your fantasies and your fears. What you think you *want* instead of what is happening right now. *Breathe.*"

—RODNEY YEE

LIMBS 5, 6 AND 7

meditation on inner calm

PRATYAHARA DHYANA DHARANA

L IMBS FIVE, SIX, AND SEVEN VENTURE INTO THE REALM of consciousness. Withdrawal of the senses (5), concentration (6), and meditation (7) form the trinity of the mind in yoga. Through these processes, we detach from the material world—which is forever throwing our sense of life's meaning into the shadows—watch the mind, and finally, attempt to still the mind.

"The process of yoga is a turning of the human soul from the egoistic state of consciousness absorbed in the outward appearances and attractions of things to a higher state in which the Transcendent and Universal can pour itself into the individual mold and transform it."

—SRI AUROBINDO

∽

"Non-attachment is *not* indifference."

—CHRISTOPHER ISHERWOOD

"Mindfulness is the energy that allows us to recognize our habit energy and prevent it from dominating us."

—THICH NHAT HANH

"Self-possessed, resolute, act
without any thought of results,
open to success or failure.
This equanimity is yoga."

—*BHAGAVAD GITA*, 2.48

"When you are climbing the ladder,
don't forget the rungs."

—SHRI SWAMI SATHYANANDA
OF VRINDAVAN

"Untrained warriors are soon killed on the battle-
field; so also persons untrained in the art of preserving their inner peace are quickly riddled by
the bullets of worry and restlessness in active life."

—PARAMAHANSA YOGANANDA (1999)

"All happiness, ordinary and sublime, is achieved by understanding and transforming our own mind."
—KATHLEEN MCDONALD

∞

"For yogis and yoginis who have cultivated detachment and are motivated by compassion, passion provides the fuel and energy for meditation upon emptiness."
—MIRANDA SHAW

∞

"The spiritual path is not strewn with roses."
—HARIDAS CHAUDHURI

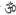
"Unhampered experience of joy which lies within comes out of simplicity."
—Swami Chidananda

"Our very way of life breeds unhappiness. We have an active and turbulent culture in which there is little peace or contentment."
—David Frawley

"Experience is . . . a tremor caused on the sea of consciousness by a gust of the wind of the ego."
—Vimala Thakar

"To control the mind with force is like putting a viper in a basket."
—MAHARAJ CHARAN SINGH

"Western laziness . . . consists of cramming our lives with compulsive activity so that there is no time at all to confront the real issues."
—SOGYAL RINPOCHE

"I heard the sea and asked,
'What language is that?'
The sea replied,
'The language of eternal questions.'

I saw the sky and asked,
'What holds the answer?'
The sky replied,
'The language of eternal silence.'"

—TAGORE

"As long as there is a 'who' asking questions, that
'who' will . . . continue to remain puzzled."

—RAMESH BALSEKAR

"It is a great mistake to think that the whole mind is what is represented by perception, intellection and will at the physical sensory level."
—SHYAM SUNDAR GOSWAMI

"Our search should not be a flight from life."
—T. K. V. DESIKACHAR

"As a painter paints pictures on a wall, the intellect goes on creating the world in the heart always."
—SWAMI BRAHMANANDA

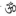
"The lotus flower has been very symbolic in the East, because the East says you should live in the world but remain untouched by it. . . . Hence the lotus flower has become a symbol of a spiritual style of living. . . . It grows from the mud in the water, and yet remains untouched."

—OSHO (1997)

"Little stones . . . pelted into the lake of consciousness should not throw the whole lake into commotion."

—PARAMAHANSA YOGANANDA

"It is easy to keep things at a distance; it is hard to be naturally beyond them."
—BUNAN

"The . . . process is to stand aside and watch the working of the divine power in yourself."
—SRI AUROBINDO

"Just sit back right now, close your eyes and train your awareness like a spotlight on the ceaseless interior parade of thoughts, emotions and memories. You believe these fluctuations are part and parcel of who you are and so cling to them tenaciously; but as I've said, all of this is what you will need to turn your back on and leave behind in order to discover and actualize your authentic self."

—RICHARD ROSEN

"When . . . consciousness is divided, not mirror-like, it becomes the mind. Mind is a broken mirror."

—BHAGWAN SHREE RAJNEESH

"We are tied to what we hate or fear. That is why, in our lives, the same problem, the same danger or difficulty, will present itself over and over again . . . as long as we . . . resist or run away from it instead of examining and solving it."

—CHRISTOPHER ISHERWOOD

"Instead of trying to erase the thoughts from the mind, it would be much better if we tried to understand the nature of the mind."

—SWAMI MUKTANANDA

"As the sages point out, wise and true seekers realize God through meditation on their own self."

—SWAMI CHIDVILASANANDA

"When the turnings of thought stop, a contem-
plative pose occurs, in which thought, like a pol-
ished crystal, is colored by what is nearby."

—PATANJALI, 41, PART 1

(CHRISTOPHER ISHERWOOD)

"It does not require a large eye to see a large mountain. The reason is that, though the eye is small, the soul which sees through it is greater and vaster than all the things which it perceives."
—MEHER BABA

"A mind that is not concentrated cannot be creative."
—RAPHAEL

"Faith is the quiet cousin of courage."
—JUDITH LASATER

"Developing inner perception does not answer all our questions but helps us to have the inner strength to live with the mystery of our questions."
—DONNA FARHI

"What is called fate or divine will is nothing other than the action of self-effort of the past."
—SWAMI VENKATESANANDA

"It is natural for thoughts to arise, just as it is natural for clouds to coalesce in the sky."
—MIRANDA SHAW

"The mind of man should be trained to love nature before he looks through the corridor of his life."
—SWAMI RAMA

"To stop your mind does not mean to stop the activities of the mind. It means your mind pervades your whole body."
—SHUNRYO SUZUKI

"The moon is one, but on agitated water it produces many reflections. Similarly ultimate reality is one, yet it appears to be many in a mind agitated by thoughts."
— MAHARAMAYANA

"Somewhere in this process, you will come face-to-face with the sudden and shocking realization that you are completely crazy. Your mind is a shrieking, gibbering madhouse on wheels barreling pell-mell down the hill, utterly out of control and hopeless. No problem. You are not crazier than you were yesterday. It has always been this way and you never noticed."

—BHANTE HENEPOLA GUNARATANA

"If you wish to see the truth, then hold no opinion for or against."

—BHAGWAN SHREE RAJNEESH

"Once you have chosen your mantram, do not change it. If you do, you will be like a person digging shallow holes in many places; you will never go deep enough to find water."

—EKNATH EASWARAN (1993)

"You need all your energy for silence of the mind, and it is only in emptiness, in complete emptiness, that a new thing can be."

—J. KRISHNAMURTI

"For by seeing and hearing one's self, and by reflecting and concentrating on one's self, one gains the knowledge of this whole world."

—*Brhadaranyaka Upanishad*, 2.4.5

"The sun has a tremendous impact upon the lives of plants, animals, and human beings. . . . Therefore, there may be a chemical basis for the thousands of years of belief . . . that to meditate and pray at sunrise and sunset is somehow more effective, more auspicious."

—Vimala McClure

"Yoga offers a set of powerful techniques for countering the tyranny of private mental chaos and moral confusion."

—BARBARA STOLER MILLER

∞

"When practicing meditation we temporarily withdraw the mind from the onslaught of daily pressures and tune into an inner oasis of calm."

—TARA FRASER

∞

"Your goal is not to battle with the mind, but to witness the mind."

—SWAMI MUKTANANDA

"Knowledge has a beginning but no end."

—GEETA S. IYENGAR

∞

"As a mighty river which when properly harnessed by dams and canals, creates a vast reservoir of water, prevents famine and provides abundant power for industry; so also the mind, when controlled, provides a reservoir of peace and generates abundant energy for human uplift."

—B. K. S. IYENGAR (1982)

∞

"Ultimately, there can be no complete healing until we have restored our primal trust in life."

—GEORG FEUERSTEIN

"The you that goes in one side of the meditation experience is not the same you that comes out the other side."

—BHANTE HENEPOLA GUNARATANA

"The purpose of all major religious traditions is not to construct big temples on the outside, but to create temples of goodness and compassion *inside*, in our hearts."

—HIS HOLINESS THE DALAI LAMA

(JOSH BARTOK)

"The mind is what it thinks. To make it true, think true."

—NISARGADATTA MAHARAJ

∞

"Consciousness . . . is compared to a flawless crystal that reflects objects in their true form. Similarly, consciousness reveals the essential, intangible core of all objects. This intuitive vision of the truth is the highest wisdom."

—SILVA, MIRA, AND SHYAM MEHTA

∞

"Meditation is not spacing-out or running away. In fact, it is being totally honest with ourselves."

—KATHLEEN MCDONALD

"Know the self as a rider in a chariot,
     and the body, as simply the chariot.
Know the intellect as the charioteer,
     and the mind, as simply the reins."

—*Katha Upanishad*, 3.3

"The process could be likened to relaxing on a riverbank and watching a fish leap out of the water, sparkle for a moment in the sunlight, then dive back in a graceful arc. There is no need to engage in a mental dialogue about the merits and demerits of the fish, emotionally react to the fish, or jump into the water to try to catch the fish. Once the fish is out of sight, it should also be out of the mind."

—Miranda Shaw

"If our mind is not at peace we shall not be happy, even in the best external conditions."
—GESHE KELSANG GYATSO

"The supreme bliss that pulsates in the wake of meditation is your pure essence."
—SWAMI MUKTANANDA

"'Just as a spider climbs up on its thread and gains freedom, so the yogin climbs towards liberation by means of the syllable OM.'"
—MAITRAYANA UPANISHAD

"Whatever the mind does, the soul has perforce
to suffer the consequences of it, because the soul
and the mind are knotted together."

—MAHARAJ CHARAN SINGH

"Meditation . . . is a practice that at once tran-
scends the dogma of religions and is the essence
of religions."

—SOGYAL RINPOCHE

"Just as the wind blowing back and forth
Controls (the movement of) a piece of cotton,
So shall I be controlled by joy,
And in this way accomplish everything."
—ACHARYA SHANTIDEVA, 6.1.76

"In meditation there is no room for coarse feelings.
The mind must be absolutely clean and purged of
all acts of hate and feigned love. Both are evils."
—SWAMI LAKSHMAN

"In meditation, mind rests. In thinking, mind moves."

—KEN MCLEOD

∞

"There is no mantra higher than meditation; no god higher than the Self; no worship is higher than inner pursuit; there is no fruit greater than contentment."

—*KULARNAVA*, 9.37

"Silence allows you to watch your mind and become aware of the thoughts that you may be acting on unconsciously. . . . We each have a unique purpose to fulfill in this life and inklings can come in those quiet moments."

—SWAMI RADHANANDA

"In meditation . . . you are . . . like an open door providing a kind of cross ventilation so that the air of divinity can move through you."

—GURUDEV SHREE CHITRABHANU

"At the beginning of every winter people are careful to install storm windows. These extra panes of glass protect their houses against the bitter winds. . . . We do something very similar to protect our minds through the practice of meditation."
—Eknath Easwaran (1992)

"The mind becomes like that on which it meditates."
—Swami Muktananda

"Goodness does not lie in dogma, not in the vanity of principle and formula. These deny love, and meditation is the flowering of love."

—J. KRISHNAMURTI

"How hard it is to control the mind!"

—SWAMI VIVEKANANDA

divine consciousness

SAMADHI

ALL YOGA, EAST TO WEST, HEAD TO TOE, POINTS TO Samadhi. *While it is not a prize to be won, it is this union which promises a release from human suffering. Our separateness, a source of pride to many, becomes our bondage to a life of ceaseless longing. The great irony of Samadhi is how easily it can become yet another thing to long for, another check on the list. The art of yoga rests in pursuit without grasping, focus without fixation, aspiration without accomplishment.*

"Samadhi culminates Yoga's eight limbs, but it is not itself the culmination of Yoga."
—GREGORY P. FIELDS

"Brahman . . . is the subtle essence that underlies the universe; and, at the same time, constitutes the innermost self or soul (atman) of each individual."
—C. SCOTT LITTLETON

"Let life be as beautiful as summer flowers
And death as beautiful as autumn leaves."
—TAGORE

"Yoga points to the truth beyond the gods of different races, nations and parochial religions."
—HARIDAS CHAUDHURI

∞

"The ultimate essence of yoga is the contact and the union between the individual consciousness and the divine consciousness."
—RAPHAEL

∞

"We all have spiritual DNA; wisdom and truth are part of our genetic structure even if we don't always access it."
—LAMA SURYA DAS

"The soul comes forward when we set aside our sense of bodily identity and recognize ourselves as an individualized portion of Divinity."
—DAVID FRAWLEY

"To one who plunges fully there is no shiver."
—SWAMI NITYANANDA

"As a light within a lantern can be seen but cannot be touched from outside, so the soul beholds the vision but cannot lay hold on it."
—RAMAKRISHNA

"I sometimes think that doubt is an even greater block to human evolution than desire and attachment."
—SOGYAL RINPOCHE

∞

"If enlightenment comes, it just comes. We should not attach to the attainment."
—SHUNRYO SUZUKI

"When I think of ages past
That have floated down the stream
Of life and love and death,
I feel how free it makes us
To pass away."

—TAGORE

∞

"While doing yoga we are more ourselves, and more than ourselves."

—VALERIE JEREMIJENKO

∞

"The eradication of the craving for personal separateness is Liberation."

—SANKARA

"That voice which is the origin of every cry and
sound is, indeed, the only Voice, the rest are
mere echoes."
— RUMI, *MASHAVI* 1:2107
(JULIET MABEL)

"As long as we live in the misperception of being
a separate entity . . . In short, we suffer."
— KEN MCLEOD

"Merely to leave darkness is not enough. Attain
to the light dispelling the darkness."
— SWAMI NITYANANDA

"In the beginning Love arose,
Which was the primal germ cell of the mind.
The seers, searching in their hearts with wisdom,
Discovered the connection of Being in Non-being."
—*RIG VEDA*, 10.129

"One must know one's own secret."
—SWAMI NITYANANDA

"From me the world streams out
And in me it dissolves,
A pot crumbles into clay,
A wave subsides into water."
—*ASHTAVAKRA GITA* (ANDREW HARVEY)

"Talk as much philosophy as you like, worship as many gods as you please, observe ceremonies and sing devotional hymns, but liberation will never come, even after a hundred eons, without realizing the Oneness."

—SANKARA

"Life is just the perpetual surprise that I exist."

—TAGORE

"Space, when limited by a jar, seems to have the difference of exterior and interior, but when the jar is broken, the space remains as one only."

—SWAMI BRAHMANANDA

"The difference between the Supreme and the individual soul is created by this sense of 'I' which
stands between."

—RAMAKRISHNA

∞

"Your divinity is incognito."

—GURUDEV SHREE CHITRABHANU

∞

"It is difficult to understand that truth is always
one. Only its expressions are new; the life-core
of truth is always the same."

—OSHO (1997)

"Reality is simply the loss of the ego."
—SHRI RAMANA MAHARSI

"Kindle the Fire of Kundalini deep
In meditation. Bring your mind and breath
Under control. Drink deep of divine love,
And you will attain the unitive state."
—*SHVETASHVATARA UPANISHAD*

"It is really one moment of looking love dead in
the eye that takes us everywhere in a flash."
—SWAMI CHETANANANDA

Om Namah Shivaya

I bow to the Lord, who is the inner self

source biographies

ARYA, PANDIT USHARBUDH, (1933–?) voiced his
knowledge of the Vedas at an early age and trav-
elled the world with his spiritual teachings.

ASHTAVAKRA GITA is an anonymous text on the
teachings of Advaita Vedanta. (Stephen Cross,
Andrew Harvey)

AUROBINDO, SRI (1872–1950) was educated in
England and returned to India to take part in the
Nationalist Movement; he then went on to devote
his life to spiritual practice.

BABA, MEHER (1894–1969) was a spiritual leader in
India who maintained silence from 1925 until his
death.

BABA, SAI was a self-proclaimed saint seen as a Divine incarnation. (Timothy Freke)

BALLENTINE, RUDOLPH is the director of the Center for Holistic Medicine in New York City.

BALSEKAR, RAMESH was an Indian scholar and author on the life of Nisargadatta Maharaj. (Timothy Freke)

BHAGAVAD GITA (the song of the Lord) is a famous yoga scripture and part of the Indian epic *Mahabharata*. (Stephen Mitchell)

BRAHMANANDA, SWAMI (1910–?) was a member of the Divine Life Society.

BRHADARANYAKA UPANISHAD, see *Upanishads*. (Patrick Olivelle)

BUHRMAN, SARASVATI is a yogic nun in the Vairagi order and teaches in Colorado.

BUNAN. (Stephen Mitchell)

BURLEY, MIKEL is a contemporary English hatha yoga scholar.

CHARAN SINGH, MAHARAJ (1916 or 17–?) was a modern saint and the author of books on Sant Mat philosophy.

CHAUDHURI, HARIDAS was educated in India and went on to become a professor of Indian philosophy in San Francisco.

CHETANANANDA, SWAMI (1948–) is the American-born director of the Nityananda Institute in Portland, Oregon.

CHIDANANDA, SWAMI (1916–?) was a disciple of Sivananda.

CHIDVILASANANDA, SWAMI (1955–) is the leader of Siddha yoga meditation in India and the West.

CHINMAYANANDA, SWAMI (1916–1993) lived in India and dedicated his life to the study of Vedanta.

CHITRABHANU, GURUDEV SHREE (1922–?) was a Jain spiritual leader who came to the United States in 1971.

CLEARY, THOMAS is a contemporary translator of Taoist literature and scholar of Eastern traditions.

COPE, STEPHEN is a psychotherapist and teaches at the Kripalu Center for Yoga and Health in Massachussetts.

DAS, LAMA SURYA is a contemporary Buddhist and author.

DESIKACHAR, T. K. V. was Krishnamacharya's son; both trained many great modern yogis.

DEVEREUX, GODFREY is a contemporary yoga instructor and creator of the dynamic yoga style.

DUNN, SAMANTHA is a contemporary yoga practitioner. (Valerie Jeremijenko)

EASWARAN, EKNATH was born in India but moved to the United States where he founded the Blue Mountain Center of Meditation.

FARHI, DONNA is a certified Iyengar yoga instructor and teaches in New Zealand, as well as internationally.

FEUERSTEIN, GEORG is a renowned scholar and author in the field of yoga.

FIELDS, GREGORY P. is an associate professor of philosophy at Southern Illinois University, Edwardsville campus.

FLICKSTEIN, MATTHEW writes about meditation. (Josh Bartok)

FOLAN, LILIAS studied under Vishnu-devananda
and brought yoga to television in the 1970s.
(Philip Self)

FRASER, TARA teaches yoga in England.

FRAWLEY, DAVID is a scholar of Vedic science and
yogic spirituality.

FROST, GAVIN and YVONNE studied and adapted
ancient Tantric teachings to Western lifestyle.

GANDHI (1869–1948) was a spiritual and political
leader at the forefront of India's Nationalist movement. (Trudy S. Settel)

GITANANDA, SWAMI (1912–?) was the founder of
the Ananda Ashram in India.

GOLDSTEIN, JOSEPH is a cofounder of the Insight Meditation Society in Massachussetts where he teaches.

GOSWAMI, SHYAM SUNDAR was a scholar of Layayoga.

GOVINDA, ANAGARIKA BRAHMACARI (1898–?) was born in Germany and then became a Buddhist of the Tibetan order.

GUNARATANA, BHANTE HENEPOLA was ordained as a Buddhist monk at the age of twelve, went on to study philosophy, and now lives and teaches in the United States. (Josh Bartok)

GURMUKH is a Kundalini yoga teacher and founder of the Goldenbridge Yoga Center in Los Angeles.

GYATSO, GESHE KELSANG (1931–) was born in
Tibet and became a meditation master. He came
to the West in 1977 and is the founder of Buddhist
centers worldwide.

HEWITT, JAMES is the author of many books
on yoga.

HIS HOLINESS THE DALAI LAMA (1935–) is the
fourteenth spiritual leader of Tibetan Buddhists.
He was their ruler until 1959 and was then exiled.
He won the Nobel Peace Prize in 1989.
(Josh Bartok, Margaret Gee)

HITTLEMAN, RICHARD is an American yoga teacher
who helped raise awareness about yoga.

IRIGARAY, LUCE is a French essayist and yoga practitioner.

ISHERWOOD, CHRISTOPHER is a Vedantic scholar and translator of many Sanskrit texts.

IYENGAR, B. K. S. (1918–) is a renowned yoga teacher who taught his method of yoga all over the world.

IYENGAR, GEETA S. (1944–) is Iyengar's daughter and was his student.

JEREMIJENKO, VALERIE is a fiction writer and ashtanga yoga practitioner, as well as an instructor.

KATAGIRI, DAININ (1928–1990) was born in Japan and came to the United Sates in 1963 where he assisted Suzuki in California; he went on to become the first abbot of the Minnesota Zen Meditation Center in Minneapolis.

KATHA UPANISHAD, see *Upanishads*. (Patrick Olivelle)

KEST, BRYAN studied with K. Pattabhi Jois and teaches yoga to packed studios in Santa Monica. (Philip Self)

KINGSLAND, KEVIN and VENIKA are teachers at the Centre for Human Communication in England.

KORNFIELD, JACK is a cofounder of the Insight Meditation Society in Massachussetts and was trained as a Buddhist monk in Southeast Asia.

KRAFSTOW, GARY studied under Desikachar and teaches Viniyoga all over the world. (Philip Self)

KRISHNA, GOPI (1903–1984) experienced Kundalini awakening and shared his experience through writing.

KRISHNAMURTI, J. (1895–1986) was a religious philosopher and teacher.

KULARNAVA is one of the most important tantras of the Kaula School. (M. P. Pandit)

LAKSHMAN, SWAMI (1907–1991) was a Kashmir Shaivite master who delivered oral teachings on self-realization. (John Hughes)

LARK, LIZ lives and teaches yoga in London.

LASATER, JUDITH teaches and trains in San Francisco. Her work focuses on yoga's therapeutic applications.

LITTLETON, C. SCOTT is a professor of anthropology at Occidental College in Los Angeles.

MAHARAJ, NISARGADATTA (1897–1981) was a seeker from India who devoted his life to spiritual work.

MAHARAMAYANA. (Timothy Freke)

MAHARSI, SHRI RAMANA (1879–1950) was a modern Indian saint who taught maha yoga. (Stephen Cross)

MAITRAYANA UPANISHAD, see Upanishads. (Anagarika Brahmacari Govinda)

MCAFEE, JOHN is the founder of the Relational Yoga Mandiram in Colorado.

MCCLURE, VIMALA is a writer and yoga teacher in Colorado.

MCDONALD, KATHLEEN was ordained as a Tibetan Buddhist nun in 1974 and teaches meditation.

MCLEOD, KEN (1948–) is a teacher in the Tibetan Buddhist tradition.

MEHTA, SILVA, MIRA, and SHYAM are practitioners and were students of B. K. S. Iyengar.

MILLER, BARBARA STOLER is a scholar of Asian cultures and translator of Sanskrit texts.

MILLER, RICHARD C. is the director of the Marin School of Yoga in California with a private practice as a therapist.

MUKTANANDA, SWAMI (1908–1982) brought his meditation technique to the United States in 1970.

NESBITT, LOIS is a contemporary yoga practitioner. (Valerie Jeremijenko)

NEWMARK, GRETCHEN ROSE is a registered dietician and yoga practitioner.

NITYANANDA, SWAMI (1897–1961) was a modern Indian saint.

OLIVELLE, PATRICK is a professor of Sanskrit and Indian religions at the University of Texas, Austin, and is the translator of many books.

OSHO (1931–1990), see Rajneesh, Bhagwan Shree.

PANDIT, M. P. (1918–?) founded the Sri Aurobindo Ashram.

PARITOSANANDA was a Tantric scholar.

PATANJALI (third century A.D.) is widely believed to have written the *Yoga Sutras*, the earliest texts to outline the eight limbs of yoga. (Christopher Isherwood, Barbara Stoler Miller)

QIU was an ancestral teacher circa the Ming Dynasty. (Thomas Cleary)

RADHA, SWAMI SIVANANDA was one of this last century's foremost women yogis.

RADHANANDA, SWAMI is the president and director of Yasodhara Ashram in Canada. Her work appears in *Ascent* magazine.

RAJNEESH, BHAGWAN SHREE (1931–) was a professor of philosophy in India and founded an ashram.

RAMA, SWAMI was an Indian scholar and yogic spiritual guide.

RAMAKRISHNA (1836–1886) was one of India's modern saints. (Stephen Cross)

RAPHAEL is a teacher in Vedanta and Western metaphysical traditions.

RAVINDRA, RAVI is a Sanskrit scholar and essayist influenced by the teachings of Krishna.

RIG VEDA (1200–900 B.C.) is the most ancient of the sacred Vedic hymns. (Andrew Harvey)

RINPOCHE, SOGYAL is a disciple of Jamyang Khyentse Choki Lodro, and went on to bring his Buddhist teachings to the West.

ROSEN, RICHARD is a yoga teacher in California and contributing editor to *Yoga Journal*.

RUMI (1207–1263), from Persia, was a Sufi poet. (also Juliet Mabel)

SALZBERG, SHARON is one of the founders of the Insight Meditation Center in Massachussetts where she teaches.

SANGHITA, SHRI DADA was an Indian saint. (Hari
Prasad Shastri)

SANKARA. (Timothy Freke)

SARLEY, ILA, and DINABADHU were founders of the
Kripalu Center for Yoga and Health and are
teachers at the Omega Institute.

SATHYANANDA OF VRINDAVAN, SHRI SWAMI is a contemporary spiritual figure. (Stephen Cross)

SCHAEFFER, RACHEL teaches yoga in New Jersey.

SCHIFFMAN, ERICH is a yoga instructor in Los
Angeles. He studied at the Krishnamurti School
in England and with masters in India.

SHANTIDEVA, ACHARYA was an ancient Indian scholar.

SHAW, MIRANDA is an assistant professor of religion at the University of Richmond.

SHVETASHVATARA UPANISHAD, see *Upanishads*. (Andrew Harvey)

SUZUKI, SHUNRYO (1905–1971) was the spiritual descendent of thirteenth-century Japanese Zen Master Dogen, and went on to make San Francisco his home.

TAGORE (1861–1941) was a modern Indian poet who won the Nobel Prize for literature in 1913. (Deepak Chopra)

THAI MONK. (Richard and Diana St. Ruth)

THAKAR, VIMALA has shared her thoughts on spiritual themes internationally.

THICH, NHAT HANH is a Vietnemese Buddhist monk and teaches mindfulness across the globe.

UPANISHADS (1300–800 B.C.) are the concluding hymns of the Vedas, the ancient sacred Hindu texts; they deal with knowledge of Brahman.

VENKATESANANDA, SWAMI (1927–1982) was a disciple of Sivananda and worked in South Africa.

VISHNU-DEVANANDA, SWAMI (1927–1993) was a disciple of Sivananda and founded the Sivananda Yoga Vedanta Centre in Montreal.

VISHWARUPANANDA was a Tantric scholar.

VIVEKANANDA, SWAMI (1863–1902) was a disciple of Ramakrishna and was largely responsible for bringing yoga to the West in the late 1800s.

WALDEN, PATRICIA studied under Iyengar and his daughter, Geeta, and is the director of the B. K. S. Iyengar Center of Greater Boston. (Philip Self)

WEST, ALISON is a contemporary yoga practitioner. (Valerie Jeremijenko)

WHEELER, KATE is a writer and former Buddhist nun.

YEE, RODNEY is the codirector of the Piedmont Yoga Studio in Oakland, California, where he teaches.

YOGANANDA, PARAMAHANSA (1893–1952) was the founder of the self-realization fellowship in California.

works cited

Arya, Pandit Usharbudh. *Philosophy of Hatha Yoga.*
Honesdale, Penn.: Himalayan International
Institute of Yoga Science and Philosophy, 1985.

Aurobindo, Sri. *The Synthesis of Yoga.* Calcutta: MP
Birla Foundation, 1988.

—. *The Yoga and Its Objects.* Calcutta: Arya
Publishing House, 1946.

Baba, Meher. *Life at Its Best.* Edited by Ivy O. Duce.
Walnut Creek, Calif.: Sufism Reoriented, 1957.

Ballentine, Rudolph. "Healing as Transformation."
Yoga International (Feb/Mar 1999): 24–31.

Bartok, Josh, ed. *Daily Wisdom: 365 Buddhist
Inspirations.* Boston: Wisdom Publications, 2001.

Brahmananda, Swami, ed. *The Philosophy of Sage Yajnavalkya*. Shivanandanagar, India: Divine Life Society, 1981.

Buhrman, Sarasvati. "Meditation Experiences." *Yoga International* (Oct/Nov 1999): 24–31.

Burley, Mikel. *Hatha-Yoga: Its Context, Theory and Practice*. Delhi: Motilal Banarsidass Publishers, 2000.

Charan Singh, Maharaj. *The Path*. Punjab, India: Radhasoami Satsang, Beas 1969.

Chaudhuri, Haridas. *Integral Yoga*. London: George Allen & Unwin, 1965.

Chetanananda, Swami. *Open Heart, Open Mind*.
Portland, Ore.: Rudra Press, 1998.

Chidananda, Swami. *Bliss Is Within*. Himalayas: A
Divine Life Society, 1991.

Chidvilasananda, Swami. *The Yoga of Discipline*.
South Fallsburg, N.Y.: SYDA Foundation, 1996.

Chinmayananda, Swami. *Self-unfoldment*. Piercy,
Calif.: Chinmaya Publications, 1992.

Chitrabhanu, Gurudev Shree. *The Psychology of
Enlightenment*. Edited by Lyssa Miller. Berkeley:
Asian Humanities Press, 1979.

Chopra, Deepak. *On the Shores of Eternity: Poems from
Tagore*. New York: Harmony Books, 1999.

Cleary, Thomas, trans. *Taoist Meditation.* Boston: Shambhala, 2000.

Cope, Stephen. *Yoga and the Quest for the True Self.* New York: Bantam, 1999.

Cross, Stephen, comp. *The Little Book of Hindu Wisdom.* Rockport, Mass.: Element, 1997.

Das, Lama Surya. *Awakening to the Sacred.* New York: Broadway, 1999.

Desikachar, T. K. V. *The Heart of Yoga.* Rochester, Vt.: Inner Traditions International, 1995.

Devereux, Godfrey. "Hatha Yoga and the Energies of Nature." *Yoga International* (Aug/Sep 1999): 30–35.

Easwaran, Eknath. *The Unstruck Bell*. Tomales, Calif.: Nilgiri Press, 1993.

—. *Your Life Is Your Message*. New York: Hyperion, 1992.

Farhi, Donna. *Yoga Mind, Body & Spirit*. New York: Henry Holt, 2000.

Feuerstein, Georg, and Stephen Bodian, eds. *Living Yoga: A Comprehensive Guide for Daily Life*. With staff of *Yoga Journal*. New York: Jeremy P. Tarcher/Perigree Books, 1993.

Fields, Gregory P. *Religious Therapeutics*. New York: State University of New York, 2001.

Fraser, Tara. *Total Yoga*. London: Thorsons, 2001.

Frawley, David. *Ayurveda and the Mind*. Twin Lakes, Wis.: Lotus Press, 1997.

Freke, Timothy, ed. *The Wisdom of the Hindu Gurus*. Boston: Journey Editions, 1998.

Frost, Gavin, and Yvonne Frost. *Tantric Yoga*. York Beach, Maine: Samuel Weiser, 1989.

Gee, Margaret, ed. *Words of Wisdom: Quotes by His Holiness the Dalai Lama*. Kansas City: Andrews McMeel Publishing, 2001.

Gitananda, Swami. *Gita Inspirations*. Pondicherry: Ananda Ashram [1972?].

Goldstein, Jack, and Jack Kornfield. *Seeking the Heart of Wisdom*. Boston: Shambhala, 2001.

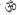

Goswami, Shyam Sundar. *Layayoga*. Boston:
    Routledge & Kegan Paul, 1980.

Govinda, Anagarika Brahmacari. *Foundations of Tibetan
    Mysticism*. New York: Samuel Weiser, 1974.

Gurmukh, Kaur Khalsa with Cathryn Michon.
    The Eight Human Talents. New York: Cliff Street
    Books, 2000.

Gyatso, Geshe Kelsang. *Essence of Vajrayana*.
    London: Tharpa Publications, 1997.

Harvey, Andrew, ed. *Teachings of the Hindu Mystics*.
    Boston: Shambhala, 2001.

Hewitt, James. *The Complete Yoga Book*. New York:
    Schocken Books, 1977.

Hittleman, Richard. *Be Young with Yoga*. Englewood Cliffs, N.J.: Prentice-Hall, 1962.

Irigaray, Luce. *Between East and West*. Translated by Stephen Pluhácek. New York: Columbia University Press, 2002.

Iyengar, B. K. S. *Light on Yoga*. New York: Schocken Books, 1965.

—. *The Concise Light on Yoga*. New York: Schocken Books, 1982.

Iyengar, Geeta S. *Yoga: A Gem for Women*. Palo Alto: Timeless Books, 1990.

Jeremijenko, Valerie, ed. *How We Live Our Yoga*. Boston: Beacon, 2001.

Katagiri, Dainin. *Returning to Silence: Zen Practice in Daily Life*. Boston: Shambhala, 1988.

Kingsland, Kevin, and Venika Kingsland. *Complete Hatha Yoga*. London: David & Charles, 1976.

Krishna, Gopi. *Living with Kundalini*. Edited by Leslie Shepard. Boston: Shambhala, 1993.

Krishnamurti, J. *Freedom, Love, and Action*. Boston: Shambhala, 2001.

Lakshman, Swami. *Self-Realization in Kashmir Shaivism*. Edited by John Hughes. Albany: State University of New York Press, 1995.

Lark, Liz. *Yoga For Life*. London: Carlton Books, 2001.

Lasater, Judith. *Living Your Yoga: Finding the Spiritual in Everyday Life*. Berkeley: Rodmell Press, 2000.

Littleton, C. Scott, ed. *The Sacred East*. London: Macmillan, 1996.

Mabel, Juliet, ed. *Rumi: A Spiritual Treasury*. New York: One World Publications, 2000.

Maharaj, Nisargadatta. *I Am That*. Bombay: Chetana, 1973.

McAfee, John. *The Secret of the Yamas*. Colorado: McAfee Publications, 2001.

McClure, Vimala. *A Woman's Guide to Tantra Yoga*. Novato, Calif.: New World Library, 1997.

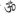
McLeod, Ken. *Wake Up to Your Life*. San Francisco: HarperSanFrancisco, 2001.

McDonald, Kathleen. *How to Meditate*. Somerville, Mass.: Wisdom Publications, 1984.

Mehta, Silva, Mira Mehta, and Shyam Mehta. *Yoga the Iyengar Way*. New York: Knopf, 1990.

Miller, Barbara Stoler. *Yoga: Discipline of Freedom: The Yoga Sutra Attributed to Patanjali*. Berkeley: University of California Press, 1996.

Miller, Richard C. "The Breath of Life." *Yoga Journal* (May/Jun 1994): 83–90; 140–142.

Mitchell, Stephen. *The Essence of Wisdom*. New York: Broadway, 1998.

—. *Bhagavad Gita*. New York: Harmony Books, 2000.

Muktananda, Swami. *Play of Consciousness*. San Francisco: Harper & Row, 1978.

—. *Meditate: Happiness Lies within You*. South Falls-burg, N.Y.: SYDA Foundation, 1999.

Newmark, Gretchen Rose. "Healing Body Image with Yoga." *Yoga Journal* (Jan/Feb 1994): 17–19, 114.

Nityananda, Swami. *Voice of the Self*. Madras: P. Ramanath Pai, 1962.

Olivelle, Patrick, ed. *Upanishads*. New York: Oxford University Press, 1996.

Osho. *India My Love*. New York: St. Martin's, 1997.

—. *Maturity*. New York: St. Martin's Griffin, 1999.

Pandit, M. P. *Gems from the Tantras*. Pondicherry: Ganesh, 1975.

Patanjali. *How to Know God: The Yoga Aphorisms of Patanjali*. Translated with commentary by Swami Prabhavananda and Christopher Isherwood. Hollywood: Vedanta Press, 1981.

Paritosananda Avadhuta, Acarya and Acarya Vishwarupananda Avadhuta, eds. *The Awakening of Self*. Calcutta: AM Publications, 1988.

Radha, Swami Sivananda. *Kundalini Yoga for the West*. Spokane, Wash.: Timeless Books, 1978.

Radhananda, Swami. "Searching for Silence."
    Ascent (Winter 2000): 7–9.

Rajneesh, Bhagwan Shree. *Neither This nor That.*
    Edited by Swami Amrit Pathik. London:
    Sheldon Press, 1975.

Rama, Swami. *Living with the Himalayan Masters:
    Spiritual Experiences of Swami Rama.* Edited by
    Swami Ajaya. Honesdale, Penn.: Himalayan
    International Institute of Yoga Science and
    Philosophy, 1978.

Ramakrishna. *The Gospel of Ramakrishna.* Edited by
    Swami Abhedananda. New York: Vedanta
    Society, 1907.

Raphael. *Essence and Purpose of Yoga.* (Translated by Kay McCarthy.) Rockport, Mass.: Element Books, 1996.

Ravindra, Ravi. *Yoga and the Teaching of Krishna.* Edited by Priscilla Murray. Wheaton, Ill.: Theosophical Publishing House, 1998.

Rinpoche, Sogyal. *The Tibetan Book of Living and Dying.* San Francisco: HarperSanFrancisco, 1992.

Rosen, Richard. "Classical Calm." *Ascent* (Summer 2000): 10–13.

Salzberg, Sharon, ed. *Lovingkindness.* Boston: Shambhala, 1995.

Sarley, Ila, and Dinabandhu Sarley. *The Essentials of Yoga.* New York: Dell Publishing, 1999.

Schaeffer, Rachel. *Yoga for Your Spiritual Muscles.* Wheaton, Ill.: Quest Books, 1998.

Schiffmann, Erich. *Yoga: The Spirit and Practice of Moving into Stillness.* New York: Pocket Books, 1996.

Self, Philip. *Yogi Bare: Naked Truth from America's Leading Yoga Teachers.* Nashville: Cypress Moon Press, 1998.

Settel, Trudy S. *The Wisdom of Gandhi.* New York: Kensington Publishing Corp., 1995.

Shantideva, Acharya. *A Guide to the Bodhisattva's Way of Life.* Translated by Stephen Batchelor. Dharamsala: Library of Tibetan Works & Archives, 1979.

Shastri, Hari Prasad, ed. *The Heart of the Eastern Mystical Teaching*. London: Shanti Sadan, 1948.

Shaw, Miranda. *Passionate Enlightenment: Women in Tantric Buddhism*. Princeton: Princeton University Press, 1994.

Sivananda Radha, Swami. "Origins of Energy: The Powerhouse." *Ascent* (Autumn 2000): 7–9.

St. Ruth, Richard, and Diana St. Ruth. *The Little Book of Buddhist Wisdom*. Rockport, Mass.: Element Books, 1997.

Suzuki, Shunryo. *Zen Mind, Beginner's Mind*. New York: Walker/Weatherhill, 1970.

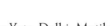
Thakar, Vimala. *Life as Yoga*. Delhi: Motilal
    Banarsidass, 1977.

Thich, Nhat Hanh. *The Heart of the Buddha's Teaching*.
    Berkeley: Parallax Press, 1998.

Venkatesananda, Swami. *The Concise Yoga Vasistha*.
    Albany, N.Y.: State University of New York
    Press, 1984.

Vishnu-devananda, Swami. *The Complete Illustrated
    Book of Yoga*. New York: Harmony Books,
    1988

Vivekananda, Swami. "Raja Yoga." *The Complete
    Works of the Swami Vivekananda*. Calcutta: Sri
    Gouranga Press, 1924.

Wheeler, Kate. "Toward a New Spiritual Ethic."
    Yoga Journal (Mar/Apr) 1994: 32–39.

Yee, Rodney, with Nina Zolotow. *Yoga: The Poetry
    of the Body*. New York: Thomas Dunne Books,
    2002.

Yogananda, Paramahansa. *Autobiography of a Yogi*.
    New York: Philosophical Library, 1946.

—. *Inner Peace*. Los Angeles: Self-Realization
    Fellowship, 1999.

ॐ

index

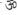

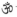

CASSANDRA POWERS practiced and worked at the Center for Yoga in Los Angeles. She currently lives and practices in New York City. She is a graduate of Brown University.